Cancer diet for the newly diagnosed:

The Ultimate Guide to a Cancer-Prevention Diet

- Dr .Zara Carmichael

Table of contents:

Chapter 1: Understanding Cancer

Sarah, a 38-year-old mother of two, was in good health and active until she learned she had breast cancer. She was terrified, overburdened, and afraid of what was ahead. She searched online for information, as many newly diagnosed cancer patients do, and was rapidly flooded with data—some of it useful, some of it contradictory, and a lot of it just plain perplexing.

Sarah's research led her to the conclusion that diet and nutrition may be highly important to her cancer treatment and recovery. She discovered that specific meals and nutrients could support healthy cell activity, enhance her immune system, and reduce inflammation. But she wasn't sure where to begin because there was so much conflicting information available.

This book fills that need. This book is for you if, like Sarah, you recently received a cancer diagnosis and are looking for advice on how to eat for your health. Here, we'll provide you with a thorough explanation of the importance of diet and nutrition in preventing and treating cancer, as well as helpful hints and recommendations for changing your diet to improve your health and well-being.

The fundamentals of cancer, the role that diet may play in both prevention and therapy, as well as the foods and nutrients that can aid in the battle against cancer, will all be covered in the subsequent chapters. We'll also provide you with a sample meal plan and some recipes for a diet that fights cancer. We'll talk about the function of particular nutrients and supplements in preventing and treating cancer, as well as typical dietary difficulties experienced by cancer patients and solutions for overcoming them.

Additionally, we'll discuss the impact of lifestyle elements in cancer prevention and management, including exercise, stress reduction, and sleep, and provide suggestions for adopting a healthy lifestyle. By the time you finish reading this book, you'll know more about how diet and lifestyle can promote your general health and well-being both before and after cancer treatment.

This book is for anyone trying to improve their health and lower their risk of developing cancer, whether they are cancer patients, caregivers, or none of the above. Let's get going.

Cancer is a complicated illness that develops when the body's cells start to grow out of control. There are numerous different cancer forms, and each has a unique set of risk factors, symptoms, and available treatments. The fundamentals of cancer, including what it is, how it arises, and how it can be treated, will be covered in this chapter.

We'll start by outlining the fundamentals of how cancer arises. When healthy cells in the body begin to grow out of control, cancer develops. Cells in the body divide and expand in a controlled manner in the normal state, but in cancer, this mechanism is flawed. Tumors are collections of aberrant cells that emerge as a result of the cells' continued division and growth.

The spread of these cells to different body regions is referred to as metastasis.

We'll then look at the various cancers and the risk factors associated with each. Certain risk factors, including age, family history, and exposure to specific chemicals or substances, might raise your risk of developing cancer. Some cancers are more frequent than others. We'll also go over the many testing and imaging techniques used to diagnose cancer.

Once cancer has been identified, there are numerous treatment choices. Surgery, radiation, chemotherapy, and targeted therapies are a few examples. We'll go through each of these therapies' mechanisms of action as well as any potential negative effects that patients might go through.

Finally, we'll talk about how diet and nutrition might help prevent and treat cancer. There is mounting evidence that specific foods and nutrients can strengthen the body's natural defenses against cancer and improve outcomes for cancer patients, even though diet alone cannot prevent or cure cancer. We'll go through the main dietary components that have been associated with both preventing and treating cancer as well as how people can alter their diets to promote their general health and wellbeing.

Readers will know more about what cancer is, how it spreads, and how to treat it at the end of this chapter. Additionally, they will be aware of the possible contribution of diet and nutrition to the prevention and treatment of cancer.

laying the groundwork for the next chapters' more thorough consideration of cancer-preventing diets and minerals.

Millions of individuals worldwide are impacted by the complex illness known as cancer. There are numerous different cancer forms, and each has a unique set of risk factors, symptoms, and available treatments. Anyone who wishes to learn more about cancer prevention, treatment, and management must have a fundamental understanding of cancer.

Cancer's progression

In order for a cell to expand and divide uncontrollably, there must be a change or mutation in the cell's DNA. Tumors are lumps or masses of these cells that can develop. Tumors come in two varieties: benign and malignant. Noncancerous and unable to metastasize to other bodily areas, benign tumors are benign growths. Malignant tumors are malignant and can metastasize, or spread to different places of the body.

Risk elements

The likelihood of acquiring cancer can be increased by a number of risk factors. Age, family history, exposure to specific chemicals or substances, smoking, drinking, an unhealthy diet, insufficient exercise, and UV radiation exposure are a few of these. It's crucial to remember that while risk factors can raise a person's odds of getting cancer, they do not guarantee that they will get the disease.

Diagnosis:

A doctor may use a number of tests and imaging procedures to diagnose cancer if the disease is suspected. A physical examination, blood tests, X-rays, CT scans, MRIs, PET scans, and biopsies are a few examples of these. During a biopsy, a small bit of tissue is taken and examined under a microscope to see if there are any cancer cells present.

Treatment:

Depending on the type and stage of cancer, patients have access to a wide range of treatment choices. Surgery, radiation therapy, chemotherapy, and targeted therapy are all possible forms of treatment. While radiation therapy uses high-energy radiation to kill cancer cells, surgery is frequently utilized to remove malignancies. While targeted therapy focuses on particular proteins or other molecules that are important in the growth and spread of cancer cells, chemotherapy uses chemicals to destroy cancer cells.

Nutrition and Diet:

There is mounting evidence that specific foods and nutrients can strengthen the body's natural defenses against cancer and improve outcomes for cancer patients, even though diet alone cannot prevent or cure cancer. A diet high in fruits, vegetables, whole grains, and lean protein sources has been linked in certain studies to a lower risk of developing certain cancers. Various nutrients, including vitamin D, omega-3 fatty acids, and antioxidants, have been linked to a range of health benefits and potential anti-cancer properties. We will go into more detail on the function of particular nutrients and foods in the following chapters.

In conclusion, Chapter 1 gives readers a fundamental overview of cancer, including how it arises, risk factors that can make the disease more likely to occur, and accessible diagnostic and therapeutic choices. The potential contribution of diet and nutrition to the prevention and management of cancer is also highlighted in this chapter, laying the groundwork for more in-depth discussions in subsequent chapters.

.

Chapter 2: The Cancer-Fighting Diet

Cancer treatment adverse effects:

A patient's ability to eat and maintain a balanced diet may be impacted by a range of adverse effects from cancer therapies. These negative effects may include oral sores, lack of appetite, nausea, vomiting, diarrhea, and changes in taste and odor. To treat these symptoms and maintain a healthy diet, cancer patients must cooperate with their medical staff.

Dietary Objectives for Cancer Patients:

Depending on the patient's diagnosis and treatment strategy, the nutrition objectives for cancer patients may change. Nutritional targets for cancer patients typically include:
Keeping a healthy weight: Losing weight is a common side effect of cancer treatment and can cause further problems. To boost their immune systems and enhance their general quality of life, cancer patients should keep a healthy weight.

Meeting nutritional needs: Because their bodies require more energy and nutrients, people with cancer may have higher nutrient requirements. In order to maintain their immune systems and encourage recovery, cancer patients must ensure that their nutritional requirements are met.

Managing side effects: As was already noted, there are a number of adverse effects that might affect a patient's capacity to consume food and keep up a healthy diet. By controlling these adverse effects, cancer patients can maintain a healthy diet and enhance their quality of life.

Malnutrition can be avoided by ensuring that the body receives enough nutrients. Due to the side effects of cancer treatments and their increased dietary requirements, cancer patients are more likely to experience malnutrition. To avoid malnutrition, cancer patients should collaborate with their medical team.

Cancer patients' dietary recommendations:

Eating a range of nutrient-dense foods, such as fruits, vegetables, whole grains, lean protein sources, and healthy fats, is advised for cancer patients. Additionally, it's critical for cancer patients to maintain their fluid intake throughout the day in order to stay hydrated.

Following are some particular dietary suggestions for cancer patients:

Eating a range of vibrant fruits and vegetables is a good way to protect your body from the harm that free radicals may do because these foods are high in antioxidants.

Selecting lean sources of protein: Protein is crucial for healing and rehabilitation.

Meats including chicken, turkey, fish, eggs, and lentils are good sources of lean protein.

Consuming whole grains can aid with digestion and avoid constipation because they are an excellent source of fiber.

Keeping away from processed and sugary foods: These can be calorie-dense and deficient in nutrients, which can result in weight gain and other health issues.

Staying hydrated requires drinking plenty of fluids, and cancer patients should strive for at least 8 glasses daily.
In conclusion, Chapter 2 stresses the value of healthy eating for cancer patients. A patient's ability to eat and maintain a balanced diet may be impacted by a range of adverse effects from cancer therapies. Maintaining a healthy weight, obtaining the nutrients

needed, controlling side effects, and avoiding starvation are among the nutrition priorities for cancer patients. Cancer patients are advised to eat a range of nutrient-dense foods, pick lean protein sources, consume whole grains, remain hydrated, and stay away from processed and sugary foods.

The chapter continues by talking about how different foods might help cancer sufferers maintain their health. Cancer patients may need to eat more protein than usual to fulfill their body's needs since protein is crucial for healing and recovery.

The necessity of carbohydrates, which give the body energy, is again emphasized in this chapter. Instead of simple carbs, which are present in processed foods and can cause blood sugar increases, pick complex carbohydrates, such as those in whole grains.

The necessity of dietary good fats is also covered in this chapter. Including good fats in the diet can really assist cancer patients maintain a healthy weight and meet their body's needs, despite the fact that this may seem paradoxical. Foods like avocados, almonds, seeds, and olive oil include healthy fats.

The chapter discusses individual nutrients and offers helpful advice for cancer patients and their caregivers on how to maintain a healthy diet. For instance, the chapter advises cancer patients to consume modest, frequent meals throughout the day to treat their morning sickness and other symptoms. In order to add more nutrients to the diet, it also advises including wholesome snacks like fruit and nut bars or vegetable sticks with hummus.

The importance of collaborating with a qualified dietitian to create a customized nutrition plan is covered in the chapter's final section. A certified dietician can assist cancer patients and those who are caring for them in understanding their particular nutritional requirements, controlling their symptoms, and creating a plan that fits their lifestyle.

Chapter 3: The Function of Nutrition in the Prevention and Treatment of Cancer

Important Nutrients for the Treatment and Prevention of Cancer:

In order to prevent and treat cancer, nutrients are essential. By giving the body the nutrition it needs to assist DNA repair mechanisms and maintain a healthy immune system, a balanced and healthy diet can help lower the risk of cancer. Additionally, as will be covered below, some foods have particular cancer-fighting qualities.

Free radicals are unstable chemicals that can damage DNA and cause cancer. Antioxidants help shield the body's cells from this damage. Beta-carotene, vitamin E, vitamin C, and selenium are a few examples of antioxidants.

b. Diets high in fiber have been associated with a decreased risk of several malignancies, particularly colon cancer. Fiber facilitates the passage of waste through the digestive system and stops toxic compounds from accumulating in the colon.

c. Omega-3 fatty acids: These beneficial fats have been demonstrated to have anti-inflammatory qualities and to be protective against several types of cancer. Flaxseeds, chia seeds, walnuts, and fatty seafood like salmon are sources of omega-3 fatty acids.
d. Phytochemicals: Plant substances known as phytochemicals have been found to have anti-cancer capabilities. The phytochemicals carotenoids, flavonoids, and polyphenols are examples. Whole grains, vegetables, and fruits all contain these chemicals.

How various nutrients function in the body and how to consume them:
Vitamin E can be found in nuts, seeds, and vegetable oils, whereas vitamin C can be found in citrus fruits, berries, and kiwi. Selenium is present in nuts, salmon, and whole grains, while beta-carotene is present in orange and yellow fruits and vegetables like carrots and sweet potatoes.

b. Fiber: Whole grains, fruits, vegetables, and legumes are good sources of this substance.

c. Omega-3 fatty acids: Salmon and tuna, two fatty fish, as well as flaxseeds, chia seeds, and walnuts, are good sources of omega-3 fatty acids.

d. Phytochemicals: The best phytochemical sources are fruits and vegetables. Examples include lycopene in tomatoes, sulforaphane in broccoli, and anthocyanins in berries.

The Function of Dietary Supplements in the Treatment and Prevention of Cancer: While the best method to get the nutrients needed for cancer prevention and treatment is through a healthy diet full of fruits, vegetables, whole grains, and lean protein, some people may benefit from taking dietary supplements. However, before taking any supplements, it's crucial to see your healthcare professional because some of them may conflict with cancer therapies or have unfavorable side effects.

In conclusion, a diet high in phytochemicals, omega-3 fatty acids, fiber, and antioxidants can aid in the treatment and prevention of cancer. A balanced diet that includes fruits, vegetables, whole grains, and lean protein can provide these nutrients. While taking dietary supplements may be advantageous for certain individuals, it's crucial to consult your doctor first.

Guidelines for Including Cancer-Preventive Nutrients in Your Diet:

Eat a variety of colorful fruits and vegetables. Since different fruits and vegetables have varied colors, so do the nutrients and phytochemicals they contain.

b. Opt for whole grains: Whole grains are a rich source of fiber and other vital nutrients. Examples of whole grains are brown rice, quinoa, and whole wheat bread.

Lean protein sources, such as chicken, fish, beans, and tofu, can deliver crucial nutrients without adding an excessive amount of saturated fat.

Limit your consumption of processed and red meats because they have been associated with an increased risk of developing certain malignancies.

g. Opt for healthy fats: Nuts, seeds, and avocados, which are rich in healthy fats, can offer vital nutrients and assist to lower inflammation in the body.

f. Steer clear of sugary drinks and snacks: These foods and beverages can cause weight gain and bodily inflammation, both of which raise the risk of cancer.

Final Thoughts: Both the prevention and treatment of cancer can benefit from a healthy diet rich in nutrients that fight cancer. You may lower your risk of developing cancer and improve your general health and well-being by including a range of vibrant fruits and veggies, whole grains, lean protein, and healthy fats in your diet. Talk to your healthcare physician or a qualified dietician if you have any worries or inquiries regarding your diet.

Chapter 4: Common Nutritional Obstacles for Cancer Patients

Patients who have cancer or are receiving treatment may experience a variety of nutritional difficulties. These difficulties can include nausea, taste alterations, and appetite loss, all of which can make it challenging to ingest enough nutrition. Here is a summary of these difficulties and some advice on how to handle them:

Loss of Appetite: Cancer treatments, worry, despair, or weariness associated with the disease are a few of the factors that might cause cancer patients to lose their appetite. Weight loss, weakness, and malnutrition can result from a decrease in appetite. Eating modest, frequent meals throughout the day and placing an emphasis on nutrient-dense foods are crucial for managing this.

Among the various tactics to take into account are:

consuming foods high in calories and protein, such as meat, eggs, beans, cheese, nuts, seeds, and nut butter
consuming calorie-dense drinks like milkshakes or smoothies
Including beneficial fats in meals, such as avocado or olive oil
Eating foods high in nutrients, such as leafy greens, whole grains, fruits, and veggies

Changes in Taste: Cancer therapies such as chemotherapy and radiation can affect a patient's sense of taste, causing a metallic or bitter aftertaste or even a complete loss of taste sensibility. This might make it challenging to enjoy eating, which can cause more appetite reduction and weight loss.

Some methods for coping with shifting tastes include:

experimenting with various flavors and spices to enhance the enjoyment of the meal
try meals at room temperature or cold because hot foods often have a stronger flavor or aroma
To help eliminate any metallic aftertaste, consider non-metallic cookware or plastic utensils.
using water to rinse your mouth both before and after meals
consuming foods that are sour or tart, such as pickles or lemons, can assist awaken taste receptors
Nausea:

Cancer therapy frequently causes nausea, which can make it difficult to eat or keep food down. Eat small, frequent meals throughout the day to help manage nausea, and stay away from items like greasy or fatty foods, spicy foods, and foods with overpowering aromas that can make you feel sick.

Among the various tactics to take into account are:

eating bland, starchy items such as rice, bread, or crackers
consuming transparent beverages such as water, ginger ale, or sports drinks
Consuming cold foods, as they may be less likely than hot ones to cause nausea
avoiding overly sweet or very sour foods
Ginger consumption, whether it be through food or a supplement, has been proven to be successful in lowering motion sickness.
Cancer patients may also gain from working with a licensed dietitian who can assist them in creating a personalized

nutrition plan based on their particular needs and preferences in addition to these methods.

Chapter 5: Special Considerations for Various Cancer Types

Diet can be a significant factor in both cancer prevention and treatment. But it's crucial to remember that certain cancers may call for various dietary strategies. An overview of how nutrition may affect the prevention and treatment of particular forms of cancer is provided below:

Breast cancer: Research has suggested that consuming a diet rich in fruits, vegetables, whole grains, and lean protein sources may help lower the risk of getting breast cancer. Conversely, a diet rich in processed foods and saturated fats may raise the risk of breast cancer. It's crucial for breast cancer patients to ingest adequate protein to promote recovery and preserve muscle mass.

Prostate cancer: According to research, consuming plenty of fruits, vegetables, and whole grains may help lower the risk of developing prostate cancer. Omega-3 fatty acids, which are present in fatty fish, flaxseeds, and walnuts, may also be good to consume. However, a diet rich in dairy products, processed meat, and red meat may raise the risk of carcinoma of the prostate.

Colon cancer: A diet rich in fiber, which is present in whole grains, fruits, and vegetables, may help lower the chance of developing colon cancer. Consuming calcium, which is present in dairy goods, leafy greens, and fortified foods, may also be advantageous. Red meat, processed meat, and alcohol should all be consumed in moderation because they raise the risk of colon cancer.

It's important to remember that because cancer is such a complex condition, nutrition alone cannot prevent or treat it. But maintaining a balanced diet can help lower the risk of getting cancer and enhance general well-being while receiving cancer treatment. Furthermore, it's critical for cancer patients to consult with their medical team and a trained dietitian to decide the most proper food strategy for their particular cancer type and treatment regimen.

Lung cancer: While no particular diet has been demonstrated to prevent or treat lung cancer, one high in fruits, vegetables, and whole grains may help lower the risk of getting the disease. Furthermore, eating foods high in antioxidants (such as berries, leafy greens, and nuts) may be advantageous. Protein and calories must be consumed in sufficient amounts for lung cancer patients to retain their strength and aid in healing.

Pancreatic cancer: Although there is little information on the relationship between food and pancreatic cancer, some studies have found that consuming a diet high in fruits, vegetables, and whole grains may help lower the risk of getting the disease. Furthermore, eating foods rich in antioxidants (such as berries, leafy greens, and nuts) may be advantageous. It's crucial for people receiving treatment for pancreatic cancer to eat enough calories and protein to enhance recovery and preserve muscle mass.

Ovarian cancer: Although no one diet has been shown to be effective in the prevention or treatment of ovarian cancer, a diet high in fruits, vegetables, and whole grains may help lower the risk of getting the disease. Consuming foods strong in antioxidants, such as berries, leafy greens, and nuts, may also be advantageous. It's crucial for people receiving treatment for ovarian cancer to eat enough calories and protein to help recover and preserve strength.

In conclusion, there is no one-size-fits-all diet for preventing and treating cancer, but there are some dietary patterns that may be helpful for lowering the risk of developing a particular type of cancer or assisting with treatment. To choose the best nutritional strategy for your unique needs and circumstances, it's crucial to consult a healthcare team and a qualified dietitian. A healthy diet is just one component of a holistic strategy for cancer prevention and treatment, which also includes regular exercise, stress management, and other lifestyle factors. This is also crucial to keep in mind.

Chapter 6:Lifestyle Modifications for Cancer Prevention and Management

Overview of additional lifestyle choices like exercise, stress management, and sleep that can help prevent and treat cancer
A detailed explanation of how these elements improve general health and well-being when combined with diet:

Along with a good diet, crucial lifestyle choices such as exercise, stress reduction, and sleep can all help prevent and treat cancer.

Regular exercise has been demonstrated to lower the incidence of breast, colon, and prostate cancer, among other cancers. Exercise promotes healthy immunological function, lowers insulin levels, and reduces inflammation, all of which can help prevent cancer. Exercise can also enhance general health and lower the risk of developing other chronic conditions.

The prevention and treatment of cancer both benefit from stress management. Chronic stress can compromise the immune system and worsen inflammation, both of which can aid in the growth of cancer. Deep breathing, yoga, and other stress-reduction practices have all been demonstrated to boost the immune system while reducing stress. Additionally, learning stress management techniques can enhance the overall quality of life and assist people in overcoming the difficulties of cancer treatment.

Additionally important for overall health and cancer prevention is getting adequate good sleep. Lack of sleep has been associated with an increased risk of breast and colon cancer, among other cancers. The body regenerates and repairs cells, including those that may have developed damage or cancer, while we sleep. Additionally, getting enough sleep helps maintain a healthy immune system and minimize stress.

generally, a nutritious diet and these lifestyle choices improve general health and well-being. People can lower their chance of developing cancer and treat the condition more effectively if they are diagnosed by engaging in regular exercise, learning stress management skills, and obtaining enough rest.

Aside from these lifestyle choices, there are other methods that can aid in the management and prevention of cancer. These consist of:

Avoiding tobacco: Smoking and other tobacco use are significant cancer risk factors, especially for lung, bladder, and throat cancer. Giving up smoking can greatly lower your risk of developing cancer and other chronic diseases.

Limiting alcohol intake: Heavy drinking has been associated with an increased risk of a number of cancers, including liver, colon, and breast cancer. The risk of cancer can be decreased by limiting alcohol use to moderate levels (one drink per day for women and up to two drinks per day for males).

Keeping a healthy weight: Being overweight or obese has been associated with a higher risk of developing numerous cancers, including kidney, colon, and breast cancer. Cancer and other chronic diseases can be prevented by maintaining a healthy weight with a balanced diet and frequent exercise.

Regular cancer screenings can aid in the early detection of cancer when it is most curable. According to your unique risk factors, discuss the timing of cancer screenings with your doctor.

Finally, cancer prevention and management is a multifaceted approach that includes a variety of lifestyle factors, such as a healthy diet, regular exercise, stress management, and enough sleep, in addition to quitting smoking, consuming alcohol in moderation, maintaining a healthy weight, and getting regular cancer screenings. By implementing these techniques into your everyday routine, you can lessen your risk of developing cancer and enhance your general health and well-being.

In Conclusion:

Although receiving a cancer diagnosis can be difficult and life-altering, it's vital to keep in mind that there are many things you can do to assist manage the illness. Your food is one of the most effective weapons you have. You may boost your body's natural defenses and raise your chances of a successful outcome by making healthy decisions and placing an emphasis on foods that are known to have cancer-fighting capabilities.

We have looked at a variety of nutritional approaches for cancer patients throughout this book. There are various actions you can take to optimize your diet for cancer prevention and treatment, from consuming more fresh fruits and vegetables to consuming less processed food.

We've also talked about the value of maintaining a healthy weight, being hydrated, and abstaining from alcohol and tobacco.

It's crucial to keep in mind that there isn't a single diet that works for all cancer sufferers. Because each person is different, what works for one person might not work for another. However, you may actively participate in your own care and increase your chances of recovery by consulting with your medical team and making educated dietary decisions.

Above all, it's critical to have a proactive and positive attitude as you navigate your cancer journey. Although diet is only one component of cancer prevention and treatment, it is a potent weapon that may help you feel more in control and equip your body with the resources it needs to combat this difficult condition. You can beat cancer and come out the other side stronger, healthier, and more resilient than ever before with the proper attitude and the correct techniques.